MELT YOUR PAIN AWAY

The Beginner's Guide to the MELT Method of Pain Relief

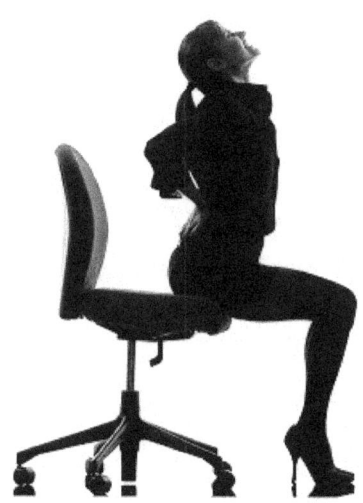

Table of Contents

Introduction

Pain affects everyone. Over time, pain restricts movement and affects mood and energy.

You do not need to live with pain. You *can* do something about it.

Read this book and discover the revolutionary method known as MELT. This method effectively deals with pain without any fancy gadgets or time-consuming exercises.

Find out what MELT is and what it can do for you. You will be amazed at how much difference MELT can make in your body and in your life.

Chapter 1: Understanding Pain

Pain is the body's way of communicating that something is wrong. Muscle pains are among the most commonly reported pain. Pain may be due to stress, overuse, improper body mechanics and fatigue. Drugs to relieve pain can only do so much and the effects often wear off sooner than desired. Long term use of pain killers is bad for the health and can cause several health problems such as abnormal bleeding and stomach ulcers.

A revolutionary, self-treatment method was developed to deal with pain. It effectively relieves chronic pain without the need for drugs or surgery. It only takes a few minutes each day to provide long-lasting relief of pain. This method is called the MELT method. MELT means Myofascial Energetic Length Technique. This technique was developed by Sue Hitzmann, which aims to restore the supportive function of the body's connective tissues particularly in the muscles, bones and skin. By restoring and enhancing the function of the connective tissues, chronic pain is eliminated, muscle and bone performance is improved, and stress is decreased. Accumulated stress comes from repetitive movements such as sitting, standing and lifting related to everyday life.

Everyday movements can cause strain on the muscle and bones, which can accumulate and cause chronic pain. People spend hours doing repetitive movements, using certain muscle groups and neglecting others. These movements include typing on computers, tapping on screens, sitting down for desk jobs, walking, standing, bending, and lifting.

All these can cause stress on specific muscle groups. This can create fatigue on the muscles and result in chronic pain.

The latest research has shown that a pain-free life is now possible. In order to achieve a life free of pain, the body has to achieve balance within the nervous system. The connective tissues should also be kept healthy. Both the nervous system and the connective tissues are directly involved in the development of pain.

More on Pain

Pain, especially those that involve the joints, bones and muscles, is a cumulative effect of several factors, which include the following:

- Years of poor body posture
- Poor body mechanics such as improper lifting and/or carrying heavy objects
- Excess body weight, which adds strain on the lower back and knees
- Congenital conditions that affect spinal and bone structure, such as abnormal curvature of the spine
- Traumatic injuries
- Frequent wearing of high heels
- Poorly fitting shoes

- Sleeping on a mattress that provides poor support

- Degenerative changes related to the aging process

MELT is a combination of neurofascial science and of applied therapy. It is designed to help people deal with chronic pain. It also has some anti-aging benefits and can improve overall health.

Chapter 2: Get to Know the MELT Method

MELT is designed for anyone and everyone. It promotes overall wellness, with some anti-aging benefits.

Who can practice MELT?

This method is often recommended for people who are in their 40s and older because it helps them live an active lifestyle and keeps them mobile and independent.

MELT is also good for athletes and younger adults because it helps in maintaining a toned and fit body. It also helps in achieving optimal performance but without the accompanying wear and tear of most workouts.

Pregnant women can use the MELT method to relieve common pain related to pregnancy, such as lower back pains due to the growing uterus.

Injured and post-surgical patients can also benefit from MELT. It can help reduce the pain related to their conditions. People with chronic pain, limited mobility and knee or hip replacements can use the MELT method to improve their conditions. It helps to promote better range of motion in the joints, relieve the accompanying bone and muscle pain and improve overall mobility. This is also good for people who have bone disorders, such as arthritis, because it promotes better joint movement.

MELT is also perfect for people who are overweight and out of shape, and is also a good start for people with a sedentary lifestyle to get some good exercise. This can also be used as a warm up exercise for any workout program.

So, as you can see, MELT can be used by just about anyone who wants to live pain free and be healthy.

The Benefits of MELT

There are several benefits that can result from practicing the MELT method. The primary benefit is a strong and more flexible body. Good posture is also achieved from the practice.

Practicing MELT can improve the following:

- Posture

- Flexibility

- Mobility

- Range of motion

- Sleep

- Digestion

- Overall well-being

- Improved mood and energy

Practicing MELT can also reduce the following symptoms related to other health conditions:

- Muscle and bone aches and pains

- Muscle tension

- Headaches

- Risk of injury, if done prior to any exercise program

MELT can also help in reducing wrinkles and cellulites in the body. It also has great overall anti-aging effect on the body.

How MELT Works

Stress creates tension within the body. Stress can be physical, emotional, mental or environmental. Physical stress can come from daily activities such as working in the office, running marathons and engaging in sports activities. It can also come from simple tasks such as carrying heavy bags and gadgets (e.g. laptops), carrying babies and children and even shopping.

Emotional and mental stress can come from daily worries, concerns and anxiety. Environmental stress can come from environmental toxins and smoke. Stress can also come from processed foods and medications.

All this stress can accumulate and become trapped in the body. This will cause tension to build up within the body's connective tissues. These are tissues that surround the muscle, joints, nerves and bones. Connective tissues are also found within every organ in the body. Trapped stress within the connective tissues results in tissue dehydration and damage. Damaged connective tissues result in poor mobility, stiffness and pains. Low back and neck pain are common. Problems arising from damaged connective tissues include headaches, digestive problems and insomnia. Development of other chronic health problems and accelerated aging process also inevitably results from damaged connective tissues.

By hydrating the connective tissues and removing the trapped stress, health is restored. Healthy connective tissues are able to function fully and prevent the abovementioned health problems.

MELT helps to keep the connective tissues in optimal health. It also helps in keeping the nervous system balanced and in optimal health. The nervous system plays a major role in chronic pain development. By keeping these structures healthy, MELT can help rejuvenate and ease the tension within these tissues.

What Makes MELT different from other pain relief methods?

MELT is different from physical therapy, Pilates®, yoga and Feldenkrais®. These methods help in promoting flexibility and in achieving proper body posture and spinal alignment. These practices focus on the musculoskeletal system. MELT is different from these because MELT specifically targets the neurofascial system. This system involves the connective and nervous tissues.

MELT includes precise and easy-to-follow techniques with the use of specialized yet simple equipment like small balls and soft body rollers. The techniques are aimed to promote rehydration of the connective tissues. This results in making the tissues more supportive and allows the release of trapped stress and tension within the muscles and nerve tissues. In simplest terms, MELT is similar to getting a full body massage, but the effects go much deeper into the tissues and the effects last much longer.

When to practice MELT

MELT is recommended to be practiced at least 15 minutes a day, three times per week. It is also OK to practice the techniques on a daily basis.

The techniques are also recommended for use prior to engaging in strength training. MELT helps in improving muscle performance during the training sessions.

It is also recommended to perform MELT after a cardio workout. It will help in relieving stiffness and compression in the joints.

Chapter 3: The MELT Method

MELT is basically a self-treatment technique designed to provide relief from chronic pain. It also facilitates healing from injuries. It also promotes health by eliminating the negative effects of lifestyle such as toxins and stress buildup.

The techniques were developed by Sue Hitzmann, renowned educator in somatic movement and a manual therapist. The techniques were reviewed by several international experts. The reviews gave further credence to MELT and recognized that the techniques are based on proven scientific principles.

MELT techniques were designed to remove the stress accumulating in the body. Stress includes physical and emotional stress from physical, emotional, mental and environmental sources. Stuck stress in the body tends to accumulate within the connective tissues, reducing the flexibility and function of the tissues they connect. The connective tissues are less able to contract and expand according the organ functions. In effect, they restrict movement, which results in pain and poor organ function. By removing stuck stress, the organs are able to fully contract and expand in accordance to their functioning.

MELT is also designed to promote hydration to the connective tissues. Dehydrated connective tissues are also unable to contract and expand, restricting movement and function of the connected organs. It shrivels up and pulls the organs tight. By restoring good hydration, the connective tissues plump up and become more elastic. This results in better function of the organs connected to hydrate connective tissues.

MELT is easy to learn and incorporate in daily life. It does not need a lot of space to perform. It also does not take up a lot of time to do. Some exercises only take as much as 3 minutes.

Instant relief is experienced after performing the exercises for the first time. More frequent performances of the exercises provide longer lasting relief. It also promotes better posture and flexibility.

Precautions

As with any other exercise, some precautions need to be exercised in order to ensure safety and prevent injuries. These precautions mainly prevent the overstimulation of connective tissues during the exercises.

- Apply tolerable pressure and keep it constant.

- For people over age 65, use additional support when doing the exercises.

- Limit the length of time lying directly on the roller if you're suffering from bone degenerative diseases such as osteoporosis and osteopenia. It is recommended to use the softer roller, which comes in a pink color.

- Use the blue or green roller if there are no bone problems or injuries. This is the OPTP Pro-roller.

- Pink rollers are used on areas that need reduced pressure. These are areas that have greater restrictions such as areas with injuries.

- Perform back MELT with a maximum of 8 to 10 minutes. Reassess after reaching this time limit and rest for 1 to 2 minutes before repeating the back exercises.

MELT is based on the 4Rs. These are reconnect, rebalance, rehydrate and release.

Chapter 4: Treatment Techniques and Materials for the MELT Method

The cornerstone of the MELT method is assessing the self. Determine the body's current state and needs. This is the most important thing to do before and after doing any of the MELT techniques.

Treatment techniques in MELT combine several methods to address the different health concerns. To reiterate, these techniques are categorized into the 4Rs of MELT, which are: Reconnect, Rebalance, Rehydrate and Release.

Reconnect

The Reconnect method is designed to reduce the stress in the body it also heightens the body's senses and improves the connection between the mind and the body. Simply put, it ensures that the nervous system is quieted down.

In the Reconnect stage, the person identifies the areas that need improvement and change. It means reconnecting or being attuned to the body. Lasting and comprehensive change is only achieved when the fundamental needs are addressed.

Rebalance

The rebalance stage is all about placing more attention to the different body organs. Focus is given to the neurocore, autonomic nervous system and the diaphragm. The techniques used in this stage prevent and decrease body pain of all types while maintaining the optimum functioning of the organs.

Rebalance techniques contacts and expands the diaphragm's range of movement in a three-dimensional direction. This is an important technique designed to reduce or prevent body pain. Rebalance also helps in promoting and maintaining organ function at its optimum level.

The neurocore system is also addressed in the Rebalance technique. This step will bring balance to the entire body. It also provides support to the gut and stability to the spine. Imbalance in the neurocore system is one of the common causes of pain in the back, paunchiness in the lower abdomen and gut problems, among others. Other core exercises do not provide enough attention to the neurocore like MELT does. MELT techniques restore the balance and optimum function of the neurocore system.

Another effect of the MELT Rebalance technique is distressing the autonomic nervous system. This system is the body's autopilot system. It provides stability to the body outside of the conscious control.

Rehydrate

The Rehydrate techniques in MELT are aimed at restoring good hydration within connective tissues and easing the tension stuck within the body. The techniques are designed to keep the body responsive and well hydrated.

Dehydration of the body's connective tissues causes toxicity, joint aches, poor posture, body pain, muscle misuse cellulites and wrinkles. It also increases the stress load of the body and the mind. Dehydration can be caused by repetitive activities, exercise and aging. MELT has special techniques that stimulate the receptors in the connective tissues. This will restore the connective tissues' hydration. In effect, this will result in keeping the body more responsive and more ready for the day's activities.

Release

The Release techniques relieve compression in the joints. Joint compression causes chronic pain, discomfort and inflammation. By decompressing the joints, the body becomes pain-free, allowing for a more active lifestyle. Particular attention is given to the neck, lower back and the joints in the hands, spine and feet.

Materials Used

MELT uses foam rollers specially designed for the different MELT techniques. Soft balls for the hand and feet are also used in some of the MELT exercises.

The soft body rollers are designed to stimulate the connective tissues and promote hydration and decompression. Techniques using the rollers aim to bring back optimum hydration to the connective tissues. They also lengthen the connective tissues. The rollers are also designed to help rebalance the body's nervous system, promote detoxification, speed up the body's healing process, decompress the lower back and the neck area, improve the stability of the body's core, promote joint mobilization, increase joint flexibility and stimulate the function of the different organs.

Rollers offer gentle decompression and compression, without adding discomfort to the targeted areas. Rollers are 36 inches long and 6 inches in diameter. If you're not too sure whether you should buy rollers right away, you can actually come up with substitutes. For one, you could use a towel – simply roll it into the right thickness (and if possible, length). If you have other exercise rollers at home, you could use them for MELT by wrapping them in soft cloth.

Chapter 5: MELT Method for the Neck

Neck pain is one of the most common pains that people consistently suffer from on a daily basis. It is often caused by poor posture and daily activities. Sitting all day working at a desk or in front of a computer is one of the most common causes of neck pain.

One effective method is using MELT to treat neck pain without the need for medications. A neck release sequence is used to promote relief.

Neck Turn Assessment:

Lie on the back with the palms facing up, the arms and legs are extended. Turn the head to the left and to the right. Then as the head is turned, take note of the following:

- Does the head move more to the left or to the right?

- Is there pain when reaching the head's end of the head's range of motion?

- Do the shoulders need to move around in order to move the head?

These would be the basis of comparison at the end of the exercise.

Base of skull shearing

1. Take roller and place behind base of skull, just below the hairline. This position maintains consistent pressure on top of the roller. To check if the roller is positioned correctly, look up at the ceiling then

slowly turn the head left to right. The roller should stay in place while the head turns. If not, readjust and keep the nose lifted and keep consistent pressure.

2. Once consistent pressure is ensured, move the head towards the right and begin the shearing.

3. Make small circular motions with the head, concentrating on small local areas within the area. It is more like making small nods. This motion will create the shear force. Shearing restores fluid state of the connective tissues in the body.

4. Pause and take a focus breath.

5. Repeat the process on the other side. Slow consistent pressure in one local region allows time for tissues to adapt. Pause after creating shear force.

6. When shear force is created, it produces fluid exchange within the base of the skull. This fluid will be used to decompress the neck.

7. Move the roller up the head about ½ inch so that the no part of the neck is touching the roller.

8. Slowly nod downwards while sustaining consistent pressure on top of the roller. Return head back up the roller. Keep movements small and slow. Take regular breaths during the movements and remember to maintain pressure on top of the roller.

9. Repeat the step 5 to 6 times.

10 Roll the head back to the center of the roller. Take one final nod and a focus breath.

11 Reassess the neck turn.

12 Remove the roller and lie flat on the back, palms up, arms and legs extended.

Results: Notice that when turning the head right to left, there is increased range, decreased pain and shoulders do not need to move much.

Chapter 6: MELT Method to Blast Cellulites

MELT can also melt fats and cellulites. The thigh area is one of the toughest areas to slim down. It is also one of the most prone to develop cellulites. MELT has the solution to this problem area. There are 3 techniques that can be performed for this goal.

Back Thigh Shear

This first move focuses on the cellulites at the back of the thigh.

1. Lie flat on your back.

2. Place the roller under the upper thighs right below the area where the thighs and the lower curve of the buttocks meet. Extend the legs in front of you.

3. Drag the legs slowly towards each other, then slowly apart. This movement should look as if doing jumping jacks or making snow angels. This targets the back of the thighs.

4. Repeat the previous step for 8 to 10 times. Pause and take 2 focus breaths.

5. Move the roller downwards, towards the middle of the thigh. Repeat step three, 8 to 10 times. Pause and take 2 focus breaths.

6. Move the roller downwards and position it just above the back of the knee. Repeat step three for 8 to 10 times. Pause and take 2 focus breaths.

Inner Thigh Glide and Shear

This second move addresses cellulites from the inner thigh by creating shear force.

1. Lie on the right side of the body. Place the roller in front of the body. Rest the head on the right arm.

2. Rest the left calf and the knee across the top of the roller. Bend the knee to position the rest of the lower leg on top of the roller. The inner arch of the left foot should rest on the end of the roller.

3. Roll the body forward, towards the roller, to bring the knee 1 inch beyond the roller. Straighten the left leg until it is perpendicular to the body.

4. Move the body slightly forward then backward. This movement should cause the extended left leg to glide over the roller. The roller should move on a small area of the inner thigh region.

5. Perform step four 8 to 10 times. Pause and take 2 focus (deep) breaths.

6. Raise the leg and bend then straighten the knee. Keep the knee on top of the roller at all times. Do this 3 times to stimulate the cells of the inner thighs.

7. Repeat the entire process with the other leg.

Rinsing the Inner and Back Thigh

Rinse is a MELT term that means a compression technique performed in one direction. This helps in moving the fluids throughout the connective tissue.

1. Sit on the floor.

2. Position the roller under the right inner thigh, just above the knee area. Straighten the right leg in front of you.

3. Use the left leg for support. Bend the left knee to provide better support.

4. Slowly "rinse up" the inner thigh. Move the body forward to move the roller slowly upwards. It should roll towards the upper inner thigh.

5. Once the roller is at the top of the inner thigh, slowly rotate the leg until the back of the thigh is on top of the roller. Pause and take 2 focus breaths. "Rinse down" the back of the thigh by moving the body backwards to move the roller down to the area just above the knee.

6. Repeat steps four and five 6 to 8 times.

7. Maintain consistent pressure on the roller all throughout the "rinsing" process. Pause and take 2 focus breaths with each pass. Repeat the process with the other leg.

Chapter 7: The Three Minute Hand MELT Treatment

The hand is a busy limb. A lot of everyday activities depend on the hand to carry them out. MELT has something for the hand in order to relieve pain from fatigue caused by constant use. This can be done at any time, at the desk or table while at work or on the floor.

Hand Grip Assessment

Before starting the MELT Hand Treatment, perform assessment on the hands. Hold the soft ball in one hand. Squeeze the ball about 3 to 4 times. Do this with the other hand. Take note for pain when gripping the ball. Also, take note if the grip is equal in both hands.

MELT Hand Treatment

1. Place the ball on the desk, table or floor. Place the right hand over the ball.

2. Position the ball at the base of the palm.

3. Move the ball between the mounds at the base of the palms.

4. Position the soft ball under the thumb pad. This is where most of the trapped stress in the hands is located. Roll the ball under the thumb pad, creating small circles. Take deep breaths while performing this step.

5. Rinse the generated fluids towards the neck. Rinse by rolling the soft ball from under the palm towards the forearm and the elbows in a single direction.

6. To end, place the right hand on the desk, table or floor, palm facing downward (towards the desk, etc.). Place the soft ball over the back of the right hand. With the left hand, roll the softball all over the back of the right hand, then roll in between the fingers, from the knuckles to the nail. Roll the ball in one direction, and avoid moving back and forth.

7. Repeat with the other hand.

Results: Reassess the hands by squeezing the soft ball again. Notice that there is less pain and the grip is stronger, requiring less effort. Also, the grip may be more equal.

Chapter 8: The Three Minute MELT Foot Treatment

The feet are among the hardest working and most neglected parts of the body. Stress can come from walking, standing, climbing stairs and driving, among other activities. Shoes are also sources of stress on the feet. Ill-fitting shoes, shoes without much support and high heels all contribute to stress and pain in the feet. MELT has a 3-minute treatment exercise to relieve and rejuvenate the feet.

Foot Assessment

1. Stand with the feet apart, about hip-width part.

2. Close the eyes. Use the body sense to pay attention to the feet.

3. Notice if there is equal weight bearing on the feet. Or, if there is more weight on one of the feet.

4. Still using the body sense, pay attention to the legs. Focus also on the joints of the hips, knees and ankles. Notice if the legs are tense and if the joints are stiff and painful.

Three Minute Foot MELT Treatment

1. Place the right foot on the football, over the inner arch.

2. Gently shift the weight of the body onto the football. This will create pressure on the ball.

3. Bend the knees and slowly move the body around. Maintain constant pressure all through this MELT.

4. Step backward using the left foot. Shift the body weight on this foot.

5. Move the football towards the front of the right heel. Move the body in order to apply tolerable pressure on the front of the heel. Slowly move the football side to side on this area while slowly moving the ball towards the back of the heel. Then reverse the movement back to the front of the heel.

6. Once the football is back to the front of the heel, increase the pressure on the ball. Move the right foot from left to right. But the ball should remain steady. This would cause the fluids to get moving throughout the foot.

7. Next, position the football directly under the knuckle of the big toe. Apply consistent and tolerable pressure while pressing the football towards the heel. Do this in only one direction. The movement would be from under the knuckles of the toes down towards the heel. Work the ball until the area of small toe is done.

8. Pause and take 2 focus breaths after working one knuckle area.

9. Repeat with the other foot.

10. Reassess the feet. Notice the improvement in the weight-bearing of both feet and the release of the tension, pain and stiffness along the leg and in the joints.

Chapter 9: The Three Minute Rebalance Sequence

This MELT is designed to improve the balance in the body, provide support to the gut and improve the stability of the spine. It also helps in improving the quality of sleep and restore energy and vitality to the body.

Start by assessing the body.

1. Lie flat on your back on the floor.

2. The palms are facing up.

3. The legs and arms are extended.

4. Use the body sense to assess the following:

   - Are your shoulders pushing against the floor? Is this on one or both shoulder blades?

   - Pay attention to the middle portion of the back. Is it on or off the floor?

   - Pay attention to the entire body. Are the right and left sides balanced? Is one side feeling heavier and longer?

Quick Rebalance Sequence

1. Lie on the roller. Position the roller so that it supports the entire back, from head to tail bone.

2. Bend the knees and place the feet flat on the floor.

3. Rock the body from left to right. Do this for 30 seconds.

4. Tuck then tilt the pelvis to keep the ribs from moving. Breathe into the length of the body by doing the following:

   - Place the hands on the chest and the belly. Take 2 focus breaths.

   - Place the hands on the sides of the ribs and take 2 focus breaths.

   - Place the hands on the collarbone and take 2 focus breaths.

   - Place the hands on the pelvis and take 2 focus breaths.

5. Place both hands on the belly and take focus breaths into all of the 6 sides of the torso (described above). When exhaling, make a "shhh" sound. Sense the gentle contraction, which stabilizes the spine and protects the organs with each breath. Do this 3 to 4 times.

6. Straighten the right leg and slide the right part of the body off the roller. Start rolling off with the pelvis, then the ribs and the head.

7. Reassess. Notice that the shoulders no longer dig into the floor and both sides of the body feel equal.

Conclusion

Thank you for downloading and reading this book. I hope it was able to help you understand that there is more to life than living with pain. And pain medications are not the only option of pain relief.

MELT is safe and the techniques are backed by scientific research.

Purchase MELT equipment now and start performing MELT today. Live a pain-free life today.

Again, thank you for downloading this book and if it helped you in any way, please leave me a nice review at Amazon. I would really appreciate it., Melinda.

About the Author

Melinda is an Amazon best selling author and mom of three

She is an avid cook, soapmaker, crocheter, loomer, and has written several books on these subjects under the "Home Life Series", all of which are available from Amazon and other fine stores in paperback and e-book format.

Melinda lives with her husband, 3 children 2 dogs, a cat, and a yellow bellied turtle in Swanville, Maine

Other books by Melinda Rolf

African Black Soap

Prep Freeze Serve

Prep Freeze Serve Chicken

Crockpot Recipes

How to Make Natural Handmade Soap

Rainbow Loom for Beginners

The Superfood Power Smoothie Book

Lessons in Clean Eating

Inside Crochet: Everything You Need to Know

The Raw Deal: The Benefits of a Raw Food Diet

Available at Amazon and other fine stores in paperback and e-book

For more about me, please visit my website at www.melindarolf.com

www.ingramcontent.com/pod-product-compliance
Lightning Source LLC
Chambersburg PA
CBHW071359310526
45790CB00019B/1652